Your Baby— Gift of God

by
Elizabeth Hambrick-Stowe

The Pilgrim Press
Cleveland, Ohio

The Pilgrim Press, Cleveland, Ohio 44115

© 1985 The Pilgrim Press

The following versions of the Bible have been quoted: KLV—*King James Version.* NEB— *The New English Bible,* © The Delegates of the Oxford University Press and The Syndics of the Cambridge University Press, 1961, 1970. Reprinted by permission. RSV—*Revised Standard Version of the Bible,* copyright 1946, 1952 and ©1971, 1973 by the Division of Christian Education, National Council of Churches. Used by permission. TEV—*Good News Bible: The Bible in Today's English Version,* © American Bible Society, 1966, 1971, 1976. Used by permission.

The Ferris quotation is from Theodore P. Ferris, *Jesus: A Sketch of the Man,* Oxford University Press, 1953, reprinted by Forward Movement Publications, Cincinnati, Ohio, 1986, pp. 8-9. The Luther quotation is from *Martin Luther Christmas Book,* arr. Roland H. Bainton, p. 23. Philadelphia: Muhlenberg Press, 1948. The Brubaker quotation is from *A.D.* magazine, November 1980. The O'Connor sentence is from *Our Many Selves,* p. 141. New York: Harper & Row, 1971. The Leboyer sentence is from *Birth Without Violence,* p. 112. New York: Alfred A. Knopf, 1975.

Printed in the United States of America on acid-free paper

98 97 96 95 94 93 92   10 9 8 7 6 5 4

ISBN 0-8298-0549-4

Preface

How wonderful for parents is the birth of a baby! It is a mountaintop moment of life: unforgettable, pure, intense, and thrilling. Out of the months of waiting, of growth and development, of anticipation there comes—suddenly—a new, fully alive, fully human person. The fetus was a stranger. The baby, seen face to face, is a definite personality. She, or he, may be small and vulnerable. But the milestone of birth has been successfully accomplished. The baby takes his or her place in the family and in the circle of humanity. In the new life we rejoice as did the prophet Isaiah: "Unto us a child is born [Isa. 9:6, KJV]." God has given us this baby.

The time immediately after the birth is most often spent by the mother in a hospital and then at home physically recuperating. Both parents—and other family members—adjust to life with the new baby. The first flush of joy in the creative power of childbirth is fresh. To friends and family the story (of pregnancy, labor, and delivery) is told. Birth's physical exhaustion and the demands now made by the newborn also have their impact on the body and spirit of parents. Help may be too little; or attention, too much. Medical questions about the infant or about jaundice or other complications cause anxiety. Sometimes the beauty of the newborn is all-captivating. Yet fathers and mothers also find themselves wondering, what will be the future of our baby? what paths will she follow? what kind of person will he be?

The story of new life is the greatest story in the world! Let it be shared, felt, and treasured as parent and child, child and world begin life together.

An Affirmation

Life is a gift from God—the gift is good!

God has created my new child, loves my child, and has a plan for my child's life.

God creates life in partnership with women and men: divine and human life, working together, have caused my child to be born.

God's love is like our love as fathers and mothers for our new baby. We can see God's tender strong love in the story of the Hebrew people, in Jesus Christ, and in the early church. The biblical story resonates with my intimate experience of pregnancy and childbirth.

Being a parent is not easy. There are times of anxiety, fatigue, uncertainty. I feel like an amateur confronted with this little baby, whose needs and wants I cannot always identify. I will need help, a chance to cry or complain, and patience—with the baby and with myself.

The beginning of new life with my child is a new opportunity for me to treasure the mystery of life, more fully to look to God as my Source, Guide, and Goal.

My child's home will be where life's first, deepest lessons are learned. My prayer is that my child will learn faith, hope, and love from me.

The Mystery of New Life

You do not know how a pregnant woman comes to have a body and a living spirit in her womb; nor do you know how God, the maker of all things, works.
—Ecclesiastes 11:5, NEB

4

The Magnificat

Mary's Song of Joy in Pregnancy

Tell out, my soul, the greatness of the Lord,
rejoice, rejoice, my spirit, in God my saviour;
so tenderly has he looked upon his servant, humble as
she is . . .
so wonderfully has he dealt with me,
the Lord, the Mighty One.
His name is Holy;
his mercy sure from generation to generation
toward those who fear him.

—Luke 1:46-50, NEB

Prayer of Thanksgiving in God's Gift of a Child

O the depth of the riches and wisdom and knowl-
edge of God! How unsearchable are God's judgments
and how inscrutable God's ways! . . . Who has given a
gift to God that God might be repaid? For from God
and through God and to God are all things. To God be
glory for ever. Amen.

—Romans 11:33, 35-36, RSV (adapted)

The Newborn Baby Praises God

O Lord, our Lord,
how majestic is thy name in all the earth!
Thou whose glory above the heavens is chanted
by the mouths of babes and infants.

—Psalm 8:1, RSV

The Responsibility of Having a Child

Before pregnancy, I lived with my own life.
Once egg and sperm met, and the dance of creation
    began, a new life was lived in me.
For nine months it grew, according to its own
    timetable and agenda . . . regardless of mine . . . yet
    dependent on me for life . . .
Now! Born! On its own the baby breathes!
And yet, dependent still, dependent now
    for caring love.
And still I live not with my own life: for
Bone of my bone, flesh of my flesh has caught my
    soul,
    and I live with its life!

Prayer for Guidance

Loving God, feeling the responsibility of this little baby, I pray for the ability to measure up to it. Help me to find the sensitivity and confidence that I need to guide and nurture my child. Help me to feel more clearly that Christ lives in me, so that I may always remember in my responsibility that I am not alone. In Jesus' name, Amen.

Partners with God as Parents

Send Wisdom forth from the holy heavens, and from thy glorious throne bid her come down, so that she may labour at my side, and I may learn what pleases thee. For Wisdom knows and understands all things, and will guide me prudently in all I do, and guard me in her glory.

—Wisdom 9:10-11, NEB (adapted)

Thoughts on Beauty

My baby is the way she is,
  looks the way he looks:
  simply *is*—beautiful!
  whether red, or dark, or pale,
  sporting a crop of baby-fine hair or none at all,
  dimpled, large-nosed, round-faced, skinny,
  enormous (tiny) feet . . .
And we love him! We love her!
With wonder and joy we treasure each little finger,
  toe, elbow. How good it is.
How good it would be
  to take our grown-up bodies with such graciousness.
After all, our eyes, hair, build, and features were
  given,
  neither reward nor trick nor punishment . . .
Wouldn't it be good
  to take our bodies as we do our babies'—
  with wonder and acceptance?

The Wonder and Beauty of the Newborn

At birth you were endowed with princely gifts
  and resplendent in holiness.

—Psalm 110:3, NEB

Paul's Insight

There is nothing for anyone to boast of. For we are God's handiwork, created in Christ Jesus to devote ourselves to the good deeds for which God has designed us.

—Ephesians 2:10, NEB

The World's Most Beloved Birth Story

In those days a decree went out from Caesar Augustus that all the world should be enrolled. This was the first enrollment, when Quirinius was governor of Syria. And all went to be enrolled, each to his own city. And Joseph also went up from Galilee, from the city of Nazareth, to Judea, to the city of David, which is called Bethlehem, because he was of the house and lineage of David, to be enrolled with Mary, his betrothed, who was with child. And while they were there, the time came for her to be delivered. And she gave birth to her first-born son and wrapped him in swaddling cloths, and laid him in a manger, because there was no place for them in the inn. . . .

Mary kept all these things, pondering them in her heart.

—Luke 2:1-7, 19, RSV

Reflections on Jesus' Birth

It is significant that he was *born*: he did not appear, he did not suddenly descend upon the earth full-blown, full-grown, as Venus is said to have appeared out of the sea. He submitted to the discipline of growth that is implied in the incident of birth. . . . His life, like ours, was a gradual unfolding of a personality in all its power and wonder. When God comes into human life, he does not often take shortcuts. He comes by way of the paths he himself has made. And so, when Jesus came into our world, it was by way of birth.

—Theodore P. Ferris

Prayer

Jesus, the Christmas baby, thank you for coming to life in a way I can understand, especially now. As with Mary and Joseph, our time came to be delivered, to give birth, and to begin the care of our newborn baby. May I, like your mother, Mary, treasure up this time of mystery and joy in my heart. Amen.

Amazing Grace

This hymn has been rediscovered recently by people across the spectrum of denominations and doctrines. In everything that makes life complicated, we appreciate the guiding Presence that sees us through. Pregnancy, labor, delivery, birth—these especially cause us to sing God's praise!

> Amazing grace! How sweet the sound
> That liberated me!
> I once was lost, but now am found,
> Was blind, but now I see.
> Through many dangers, toils, and snares
> I have already come;
> 'Tis grace has brought me safe thus far,
> And grace will lead me home.
> —John Newton

Martin Luther, Father of Six Children:

To me, there is no greater consolation than this given humankind, that Christ became a man, a child, a babe, playing in the lap and at the breasts of this his most gracious mother. Who is there whom this sight would not comfort? . . . God places before you a babe, with whom you can take refuge. You cannot fear him, for nothing is more appealing to people than a babe.

9

Love Is a Circle

Little do children know the affection that lies in the heart of a father.

—Increase Mather, 1639-1723

I knew I would love my children long before I ever had them. I was not prepared for how much they would love me. That was one of the most unexpected gifts I've ever been given.

—Ann Brubaker

Prayer for Quietness

Loving God, so much has happened these days! I've been down in the depths and up on the heights. The long wait of pregnancy feels like a dream, now that the baby is born. I'm all excited, yet sometimes I feel anxious about what life will be like with this new child. Touch my soul, dear God, with quietness, with calmness and peace. By Jesus' spirit, Amen.

Especially for Parents of Little Babies

Practice accepting what the day brings over which you have no control.

—Elizabeth O'Connor

Jesus' Blessing

Then he took a child, set him in front of them, and put his arm round him. "Whoever receives one of these children in my name," he said, "receives me; and whoever receives me, receives not me but the One who sent me."

—Mark 9:37, NEB

Labor of Love

Labor: Work
  "The hardest work you'll ever do," said our Lamaze
  teacher.
Labor: Pain and Stress
  Tears may flow in the night.
Labor: Total Exertion
  Long have I lain still, I kept silence and held myself
  in check; now I will cry like a woman in labour.
Labor: Exhaustion
  Come unto me, all ye that labour and are heavy
  laden, and I will give you rest.
Labor: Fearful Unknown
  Now my soul is in turmoil, and what am I to say?
  Father, save me from this hour.
NO: Jesus explained, with us in the delivery
  room, laboring, nine-months-expectant:
"No, it was for this that I came to this hour," and
  although "tears may flow in the night,
Joy comes in the morning!"
For "a woman in labour is in pain because her time
has come; but when the child is born she forgets the
anguish in her joy that a human being has been born
into the world."
—Psalm 30:5, TEV; Isaiah 42:14, NEB; Matthew 11:28,
        KJV; John 12:27-28, NEB; John 16:21, NEB

Prayer After Labor

  Holy Spirit, Comforter, and Strength: through the
valley of the shadow of labor you have kept and
preserved mother and baby. I am thankful for the
assistance of those persons who helped my child to
make the risky transition from its first inner home
and to be born into the world. How glad I feel in this
work well done! Praise God! Amen.

Thoughts on Naming the Child

A good name is more to be desired than great riches.

—Proverbs 22:1, NEB

Every child has the right to a name, says the United Nations Declaration on the Rights of a Child. A name gives personal identity. In naming the newborn child, parents have a joyful obligation to their baby.

A name may be given from family lineage or ethnic heritage. It may be the name of a wise, respected, beloved friend or teacher. The name may represent to the parents a happy place or time or a pleasing sound. The baby's own appearance may suggest a fitting name. The name may be biblical or historical.

Each child should grow to feel that his or her name is special, that it was chosen with care, and that a "good name" is both a goal in life and a source of strength for living.

God Knows Us by Name

But now this is the word of the Lord,
the word of your creator, O Jacob,
of him who fashioned you, Israel:
Have no fear . . . I have called you by name
and you are my own.

—Isaiah 43:1 NEB

Prayer in Naming

Loving God, bless the name given to our baby. May she or he grow to be a person with a good name and reputation. Help me to set a good example for my child. Release in me the power that comes from bearing Christ's name, in Christian faith. Amen.

A Prayer When Worried

O God, I feel so vulnerable because of my little baby. When something is not quite right, when the nurses and doctors say, "We just want to check it out," I feel anxiety rising inside me. A few ounces of birthweight lost, a rise in jaundice, whatever the problem happens to be—I'm worried. Please help me to feel your Presence in strength and power, just as you shared the worries of anxious parents in Jesus' healing, life-giving ministry. Amen.

Child's Song

Jesus loves the little children,
  All the children of the world:
Red and yellow, black and white,
  Each is precious in his sight.
Jesus loves the little children of the world.

A Hymn for Strength in God

When you pass through deep
  waters, I am with you,
when you pass through rivers,
they will not sweep you away;
walk through fire and you will not be scorched,
through flames and they will not burn you.
For I am the Lord your God,
the Holy One of Israel, your deliverer.

—Isaiah 43:2-3, NEB

In the Maternity Ward

A maternity ward is a strange place. It is a twentieth-century invention. Before, babies were born at home, most often with the assistance of other women. Now, physicians direct the delivery, professional nurses tend the newborns. Babies are brought to their mothers at certain times for feeding. A choice must usually be made between the presence of the baby or visitors. In the nursery a glass wall separates babies from everyone; parents, grandparents, siblings, friends alike view the newest family member through the dividing glass. But the maternity experience—although strange—is usually positive.

Maternity nurses are, by and large, a pleasant caring staff to infants and families. The facilities of labor and delivery rooms aid the midwife or physician in delivering each precious new life safely. Most hospitals make a special effort to ensure a restful and celebrative maternity stay. If this birth is not the first child, the mother may not be in a hurry to leave the comfort and service provided! Finally, there is a powerful sisterhood in the grouping of new mothers, a brotherhood of new fathers.

Prayer in the Maternity Ward

Delivering God, you call your creation into life: thank you for all who act as your instruments of safe birth. For devoted physicians, midwives, nurses, each member of the hospital staff, whose energies go toward making the maternity stay a time of health, comfort, and rest, I give thanks. May they all be gladdened, strengthened, and encouraged in their work by the privilege of working with you in the miracle of new life. Amen.

Jesus and the Children

They even brought babies for him to touch. When the disciples saw them they rebuked them, but Jesus called for the children and said, "Let the little ones come to me; do not try to stop them; for the kingdom of God belongs to such as these. I tell you that whoever does not accept the kingdom of God like a child will never enter it."

—Luke 18:15-17, NEB

The Good Baby

Already, baby and world meet each other.
My baby acts by instinct to eat, sleep, stretch, cuddle,
    cry.
My baby's personality shows itself in *how* he eats,
    sleeps, stretches, cuddles, cries.
Already, people ask, "Is she a good baby?"
They mean: Does she eat quickly and well, burp, go
    back to sleep or lie quietly? They mean: Does
    the baby not have day and night mixed up?
They mean: Is the baby not a lot of bother?
Lord, guard me from judging my baby!
Lord, guard me from judging myself!
We're just getting to know each other. "Bother" is not
    "bad."
We're just getting used to each other,
    baby and me, baby and world . . .
Oh yes, the baby's very good!

Says the Creator:

Can a woman forget the infant at her breast,
or a loving mother the child of her womb? . . .
I will not forget you.

—Isaiah 49:15, NEB

A Mother's Poem to Her Eight Children

I had eight birds hatched in one nest,
Four Cocks there were, and Hens the rest,
I nursed them up with pain and care,
Nor cost, nor labor did I spare,
Till at last they felt their wing,
Mounted the Trees, and learned to sing . . .

Great was my pain when you I bred,
Great was my care, when I you fed,
Long did I keep you soft and warm,
And with my wings kept off all harm . . .

When each of you shall in your nest
Among your young ones take your rest,
In chirping language, oft them tell,
You had a Dam [mother] that loved you well,
That did what could be done for young,
And nursed you up till you were strong,
And 'fore she once would let you fly,
She showed you joy and misery;
Taught what was good and what was ill,
What would save life, and what would kill.

—Anne Bradstreet, 1656

Children Learn What They Live

If a child lives with criticism, he learns to condemn.
　　If a child lives with hostility, she learns to fight.
If a child lives with ridicule, he learns to be shy.
　　If a child lives with shame, she learns to feel guilty.
If a child lives with tolerance, he learns to be patient.
　　If a child lives with encouragement, she learns
　　confidence.
If a child lives with praise, she learns to appreciate.
　　If a child lives with fairness, he learns justice.
If a child lives with security, he learns to have faith.
　　If a child lives with approval, she learns to like
　　herself.
If a child lives with acceptance and friendship,
　　he learns to find love in the world.

Pondering the Future

> What then will this child be?
> 　　　　—Luke 1:66, RSV

What Now, Lord?

What does the baby need? What does the baby want?
Here's what I've checked: diapers, pins, air
　　bubbles, too much (or too little) clothing.
Here's what I've done: feeding (wasn't hungry),
　　rocking (still crying), patting (still awake).
Here's how the baby's feeling: miserable.
Here's how I'm feeling: miserable!
What now, Lord? Amen.

Prayer When Feeling Overburdened

Loving God, please help me when I feel over-whelmed and confused in the care of this little baby. I cannot do a good job alone for very long. Guide me toward those other family members and friends who can share the joys and the burden of nurturing this tiny, demanding person. Amen.

Starting a Pilgrimage of Life

But now we are all in all places strangers and pil-grims, travelers and sojourners, most properly hav-ing no dwelling but in this earthen tabernacle. Our dwelling is but a wandering, and our abiding but as a fleeting, and in a word our home is nowhere but in the heavens—in that house not made with hands, whose maker and builder is God, and to which all ascend who love the coming of our Lord Jesus.
—Robert Cushman, 1622

Life is a journey from birth through all the stages of life. One of the great enjoyments of being a parent is to watch this child develop from day to day. The journey is not just one of physical and emotional growth. God wants us to travel through life discover-ing more and more about what it means to be God's child. In our homes and families we progress spiritu-ally, in love with one another and with God. The goal of life is our home with Jesus in God's heavenly king-dom. Our baby is a pilgrim just setting out on this journey. May God bless us as we take the first steps together.

Paul to Timothy on His Family Heritage:

I am reminded of your sincere faith, a faith that dwelt first in your grandmother Lois and your mother Eunice and now, I am sure, dwells in you.

—2 Timothy 1:5, RSV

Prayer for the Extended Family

God of Abraham and Sarah, Isaac and Rebecca, Jacob and Rachel: Your plan for life places each child into a wider family circle: grandparents, uncles and aunts, cousins, relations by blood and affection. We thank you for the increase of our joy that comes from this circle, welcoming our baby in love. Make the time of family visits to the new baby a chance for each to express words of love to one another. Let our family be drawn more closely together in celebrating its newest life. Amen.

Jesus' Extended Family Shares the Joy of Childbirth

[The angel Gabriel said to Mary:] "Behold, your kinswoman Elizabeth in her old age has also conceived a son; and this is the sixth month with her...." In those days Mary arose and went with haste into the hill country . . . and she entered the house of Zechariah and greeted Elizabeth. . . . And Mary remained with her about three months [until the baby John was born], and returned to her home.

—Luke 1:36, 39-40, 56, RSV

Thoughts on Helpful Friends and Visitors

When Jesus was born, three wise men, or kings, came to see him and to leave rich gifts, according to the Gospel of Matthew. In this nativity story there is something familiar. Family and friends come by to see our baby. The ohs and ahs of admiration and delight spring from our reverence for new life. Cards and plants, baby items, and welcome gifts of food for family during the first days back home are symbols of ties that bind us together in faith and friendship.

The visits of the wise men and the shepherds to the infant Jesus confirmed that he would live for others, not only for his birth family. The visits, gifts, and help of our friends remind us that we are brothers and sisters, one family of humanity, and that there is a wide world of good people for the baby to discover as she or he grows. Praise God for the expressions of caring people in this special time.

At the Beginning of Life

The newborn is a mirror, reflecting our image.
—Frederick Leboyer

The Fruit of the Spirit

The fruit of the Spirit is love, joy, peace, patience, kindness, goodness, faithfulness, gentleness, self-control. . . . If we live by the Spirit, let us also walk by the Spirit.

—Galatians 5:22-23, 25, RSV

Care-taking

Then you may suck and be fed from the breasts that
    give comfort,
delighting in her plentiful milk.
For thus says the Lord:
I will send peace flowing over her like a river,
and the wealth of nations like a stream in flood;
it shall suckle you,
and you shall be carried in their arms
and dandled on their knees.
As a mother comforts her son,
so will I myself comfort you,
and you shall find comfort.

—Isaiah 66:11-13, NEB

Getting to Know You

A perspective on the never-ending tasks of baby
care was given to me by a pastor's wife, herself a
grandmother.

Although a busy person, her baby gift was a
weekly morning of child care during the first months
after our premature twins came home from the hospital. She bathed, powdered, diapered, dressed, and
rocked them, singing or talking in quiet tones. Each
necessary task, she said, is a time and occasion for
getting to know the babies—and for them to know us
by the infants' first languages of hearing and acute
sense of touch. Taking care of babies, she demon-
strated, is not *doing* a chore, but *being with* babies at
their own infant level. As Paul said of his ministry,
"To the weak I became weak, that I might win the
weak [1 Cor. 9:22, RSV]."

Prayer in Care-taking

Eternal God, in divine wisdom you have made our human babies utterly dependent on the care of adults, who ourselves lived and grew because our parents took care of us. Thank you for weaving between me and my baby the bonds of love, as we share together the tasks of daily life. Amen.

Waiting Time

In the hospital we are waiting to go home. These days between birth and homecoming are unlike any other days. So full of excitement, emotional release, and nervous anticipation. These are days of waiting.

Make the most of these days! Do not simply wait for time to pass until they say that mother and baby can leave. Wait creatively, spiritually. These are special days in which God wants to bless us as new parents. Beyond the human love that may surround us, God is with us in a tender way when we hold and feed our baby in these first days . . . and in the quiet times, when we are alone with the room curtains drawn.

If we wait for the Lord, then God who came to earth in Jesus Christ will fill us, will fill these quiet days and nights with strength for all the strenuous days and nights to come at home, so we will be equal to the tasks ahead.

Our Baby Is a Gift from God

Children are a gift from the Lord;
   they are a real blessing.
                    —Psalm 127:3, TEV

Our Family Is Gifted

Stir into flame the gift of God which is within you.

There are varieties of gifts, but the same Spirit.

Hold unfailing your love for one another, since love covers a multitude of sins. . . . As each has received a gift, employ it for one another, as good stewards of God's varied grace.
      —2 Timothy 1:6, NEB; 1 Corinthians 12:4, RSV;
                    1 Peter 4:8, 10, RSV

The Gift of Grace and Abundant Life

The free gift of God is eternal life in Christ Jesus our Lord.

But grace was given to each of us according to the measure of Christ's gift.
         —Romans 6:23, RSV; Ephesians 4:7, RSV

Thank God for These Gifts

God of grace and love, thank you for the miraculous gift of our baby. Bind us together in your saving grace through our faith in Jesus, who is your gift to us and every family of earth. Enable us as the years unfold to know the special gifts of our child. Guide us as we help our child discover these gifts and learn to use them in ways that will make life good in your sight, and to the glory of your name. Amen.

Prayer for a Christian Home

O Christ, thyself a child within an earthly home,
With heart still undefiled, thou didst to manhood
   come;
Our children bless, in every place,
That they may all behold thy face,
   And knowing thee may grow in grace.

O Spirit, who dost bind our hearts in unity,
Who teachest us to find the love from self set free,
In all our hearts such love increase,
That every home, by this release,
   May be the dwelling place of peace.

                   —F. Bland Tucker

Faith Is a Family Affair

Over and over the Bible states God's plan for life.
God offers a covenant to us and to our children, a
saving and sustaining relationship of promise. No
one is too young for God to love, preserve, and keep.
There is no reason to wait until a child is any particu-
lar age before including him or her in the family of
faith. After all, from birth we surround our newborn
with care and affection. As John said, love is not a
matter of words or talk but of action (1 John 3:18). We
show our baby, we don't *tell* the baby about, mother's
and father's love. Just so, each baby belongs in the
church. Surrounded by the care and affection of the
Christian community, the child will "grow and
become strong, filled with wisdom; and the favor of
God [Luke 2:40, RSV]."